Management of cataract in primary health care services

World Health Organization
Geneva
1990

WHO Library Cataloguing in Publication Data

Management of cataract in primary health care services.

1. Cataract   2. Cataract extraction   3. Primary health care –
organization & administration

ISBN 92 4 154408 2   (NLM Classification: WW 260)

© World Health Organization 1990

TYPESET IN INDIA
PRINTED IN ENGLAND

89/8305—Macmillan/Clays/GCW—5500

Contents

Preface

Cataract, generally defined as an opacity of the crystalline lens of the eye, is a major cause of visual impairment and blindness worldwide. This disorder, which has been documented since very early times, was recognized by the Twenty-eighth World Health Assembly in 1975[1] as one of the most important causes of avoidable blindness.

Cataract accounts for nearly half of all blindness, and is particularly common in developing countries. The grim fact is that there already exists a formidable total of some 17 million people needlessly blind from cataract. With the rapid "greying" of the population, the problem of blindness from cataract will assume even more staggering proportions in the future.

In the present state of knowledge, there is no proven means of preventing cataract or its progression to blindness. The condition is, however, amenable to surgical treatment, which, together with the optical correction of the ensuing refractive deficit, results in the restoration of vision.

In developed countries, the availability of eye care services to those blind from cataract ensures that the large majority have their sight restored. In contrast, in the developing countries, in which the majority of the cataract blind are found, there has been over the years an accumulation of unattended persons blind from cataract, resulting in what is commonly referred to as the "cataract backlog".

It has therefore become imperative that programmes for the control of blindness should include, as an important component, interventions for the surgical restoration of vision in persons blind from cataract. These should be an integral part of the primary health care system, so that most of the people who now make up the "cataract backlog" will have better access to surgical services.

---

[1] Resolution WHA28.54.

This publication contains comprehensive guidelines on the management of cataract through primary health care. It includes a review of the available information on the prevalence of blindness resulting from cataract, strategies for action against cataract, guidelines for the planning of interventions, including development of human resources and infrastructure, as well as managerial requirements for effective action.

The basic guidelines outlined in this publication, which are intended for adaptation to suit local conditions, will help to ensure intensified action against cataract and the restoration of vision to those already blind or destined to become blind from cataract in the future.

*

*　　*

The colour photographs were kindly supplied by Dr Jock Anderson, Dr Allen Foster, Professor Gordon Johnson, Dr Murray McGavin, and Dr David Yorston.

1. Clinical aspects

Definition

The term "cataract" is derived from the Latin word *cataracta*, which is in turn derived from the Greek word *kataraktes*, which means waterfall (breakdown, downrushing). Ancient practitioners probably gave this name to the condition in the belief that the liquid content of the eye was cascading down.

Defined strictly on the basis of the pathomorphological process involved, cataract is an opacification or loss of transparency in the crystalline lens of the eye. From a public health perspective, however, attention also needs to be paid to the consequences of such an opacification in terms of visual acuity.

In a large number of instances, the opacity, by virtue of its size or position, does not affect vision. In many cases, the opacity is not progressive and mere identification of such an opacity during mass eye examination surveys or clinical examination does not necessarily portend progression to blindness in the future. These considerations sometimes confound the data on cataract diagnosed during eye examinations in blindness surveys, in respect both of the actual prevalence of cataract and of the annual incidence of new cases requiring surgery. An accurate estimation of both rates is essential for determining the magnitude of the existing problem, as well as for predicting how it is likely to develop in the medium and long term. Such a prediction would make it easier to plan interventions against cataract as part of national programmes for the prevention of blindness.

Types of cataract

Cataract can be classified by age of onset (e.g., congenital, juvenile, or "senile" cataract) or by location of the opacity within the lens (e.g., cortical or nuclear). In addition, cataract may be designated as being the result of, or secondary to, other ocular diseases, systemic disorders, and genetic or environmental influences.

The type of cataract and consequent blindness that gives rise to public health problems is generally related to aging ("senile" cataract). However, congenital cataract and cataracts resulting from trauma, *inter alia*, pose special problems in management with regard to both prevention and treatment. While prevention is part of primary eye care, management of such cataracts is generally the responsibility of institutions that can provide the necessary sophisticated instrumentation often required for treatment and follow-up, and will not be described here.

Cataracts can also be classified in relation to their stage of maturity, i.e., as incipient, immature, mature or hypermature. An incipient cataract is a lens opacity that interferes with vision, if at all, to a very small extent and produces only a slight localized or generalized reduction of the red reflex. An immature cataract is a further stage of lens opacification which reduces vision to better than hand movements and in which there is a marked generalized reduction of the red reflex. A mature cataract is defined as a totally opaque lens which reduces the visual acuity to hand movements or less, and in which there is a total absence of the red reflex. Swelling of the lens may occur when a cataract has reached an advanced stage (intumescent cataract). Finally, the term *hypermature cataract* is applied to a cataractous lens that has shrunk, often with a wrinkling of the capsule. Vision is generally restricted to hand movements or less, and the red reflex is absent.

The above classification is important from a public health point of view, not only in eye examination surveys but also because of the deleterious effect that delay in surgery can have in the mature (Morganian) and hypermature stages. This has important implications for the planning of timely cataract intervention services and in assigning priorities for surgical intervention, if irreversible blinding complications are to be averted.

The pathway to blindness in cataract is generally direct and is the result of the impediment that the lens opacity poses to the entry of light beyond the pupil. However, where the lens becomes swollen (intumescent cataract) or hypermature, provoking an inflammatory or cellular (phacolytic) reaction, secondary glaucoma may supervene; if not urgently and appropriately managed, this can lead to irreversible loss of vision. Secondary glaucoma may also ensue from displacement of long-standing cataractous lenses in the very elderly, either spontaneously or often as a consequence of minor trauma.

Such dislocation may, however, be caused intentionally, as in the procedure called "couching". This ancient technique is still practised in some developing countries, often by itinerant traditional practitioners in remote rural areas not served by cataract surgical services. The procedure is very likely to produce severe complications which, more often than not, render the eye blind within a very short period of time.

Symptoms and signs

Symptoms

An opacity of the lens may be present without causing any symptoms, and may be discovered only on routine ocular examination.

A gradual and painless deterioration of vision in an older person is generally suggestive of cataract. However, other conditions, such as chronic glaucoma, macular changes in diabetes mellitus, and senile macular degeneration, need to be excluded.

One of the earliest visual disturbances with cataract is glare or intolerance of bright light, such as direct sunlight or the headlights of an oncoming motor vehicle. The amount of glare or dazzle will vary with the location and size of the opacity, those occurring in the pupillary area causing symptoms out of proportion to their size. In the early stages, the visual acuity may be normal on routine testing. As the lens opacity progresses, the quality of vision begins to suffer, with an associated fall in acuity of both distance and near vision.

However, where nuclear sclerosis predominates, an improvement in near vision may become apparent as a result of myopia of lenticular origin. Thus an individual who has hitherto required glasses for near work may find that it is possible to dispense with them. However, at the same time, the visual acuity for distance becomes impaired. Before long, the individual's activities are restricted as a result of the further progression of the opacity, and surgical removal of the lens is necessary.

Other visual disturbances include misty vision, dulling of colour sense and occasionally monocular double vision. The consequences of lens-induced uveitis and secondary glaucoma have been referred to earlier; these are heralded by severe pain and redness in the eye. This often occurs in patients who have earlier had vision restored in one eye but have ignored a long-standing cataract in the other eye.

Signs

Evidence of lowered visual acuity together with a dull or absent red reflex is suggestive of the diagnosis of cataract. However, cloudiness of the cornea or vitreous body from any cause needs to be excluded. When the cataract is more developed, a grey or white pupil is observed. In mature cataract, vision may be reduced to hand movements or even light perception. It is important to test for light projection in such eyes to exclude possible underlying disease of, or damage to, the retina or optic nerve.

The pupil in eyes with cataract is normally briskly reactive to light. This is an important clinical sign which denotes healthy retinal and optic nerve function and is predictive of a successful outcome following surgery.

2. Cataract as a public health problem

The type of cataract that constitutes a public health problem is the age-related opacification of the lens that impairs vision to such an extent that occupational pursuits or the activities of daily living are severely restricted. Such restrictions lead to economic and psychological deprivation that adversely affects the quality of life.

The growing life expectancy worldwide, and particularly in developing countries, is already leading to a rapid increase in the number of elderly people. In the current absence of proven methods for preventing or delaying the progression of human cataract, this aging of the population will lead to a phenomenal increase in the number of the cataract blind.

Age-related cataract, which is usually bilateral, is amenable to surgical treatment that is both safe and effective. Surgical output, particularly in developing countries, cannot cope even with the new cases of blindness due to cataract, leading to an inevitable "snowballing" of the number unattended. This is the public health dimension of the problem that needs to be addressed.

Prevalence

In 1984, there were an estimated 27–35 million persons blind (vision less than 3/60 in the better eye) from all causes. Of these, approximately half were blind from cataract. There are marked differences in the prevalence of cataract, related both to ethnicity and to geographical location. The percentage of cataract-related blindness in relation to the overall prevalence of blindness is given for selected countries in Table 1.

Incidence

It is estimated that there is an annual increase in the backlog of people requiring surgery of over 2 million persons newly blind

5

Table 1. Prevalence of blindness and percentage of cataract-related blindness in certain countries

Region	Population (thousands)	Prevalence of blindness (%)	Cataract-related blindness per 100 blind
Africa			
Chad	5 018	2.3[a]	48.0
Congo	1 740	0.3[a]	81.0
Gambia	643	0.7[a]	55.0
Eastern Mediterranean			
Saudi Arabia	11 542	1.5[a]	55.1
Tunisia	6 890	3.9[b]	52.4
South-East Asia			
India	800 000	1.5[b] 0.7[a]	81.0
Indonesia	150 958	1.2[a]	66.9
Nepal	14 667	0.8[a]	66.8
Thailand	49 460	1.1[a]	56.6
Western Pacific			
China	1 059 521	0.4[a,c]	57.1
Japan	116 807	0.3[b]	23.0
Philippines	51 960	1.1[a]	87.2

[a] Less than 3/60 in better eye.
[b] 6/60 or less in better eye.
[c] Limited survey.

from cataract; this is compounded by the demand for surgery at earlier stages of visual impairment in many communities, in keeping with socioeconomic development. These figures for incidence are based on prospective studies in pilot areas, which do not lend themselves to extrapolation to other areas and particularly to developing countries, and are thus subject to considerable uncertainty.

6

In any computation of the target number of people to be treated within a given time, it is necessary to take a number of factors into account, including the existing backlog, the estimated surgical output, the attrition from mortality of persons blind from cataract, and the incidence of new cases estimated from demographic data.

Methods of estimating the annual incidence of new cases of cataract blindness have been described in some countries. One such calculation takes into account the point prevalence of cataract (derived from a blindness survey), an estimated annual incidence (based on questionnaire responses during the survey), the annual rate of increase in the age cohort with cataract blindness (from demographic data), and various assumptions about death rates and surgical coverage rates.

In another country, a simpler method for calculating annual incidence in different age groups was used taking into account the prevalence of cataract blindness in the age subgroup with the highest rate, i.e., over 60 years of age, life expectancy at age of entry into the group, the number of people entering this population subgroup annually (from demographic data), and the number of years from entry into this group until death.

However, neither of these methods is easily applicable and the results of proper cohort studies must therefore be awaited before one that is both practical and reliable can be developed.

Age

Senile cataract generally occurs in persons above the age of 50 years. It is estimated that 50% of all those in the sixth decade and nearly 100% in the age group 80 years and older have some opacity. These lens opacities are not necessarily associated with visual impairment or blindness.

The prevalence of senile cataract increases with age, and this trend is clearly seen in blindness prevalence studies. It is therefore important to look at the likely demographic trends in respect of the elderly population (over 60 years) in the developing countries over the next 20–30 years. In developing countries, infant and childhood mortality are falling and people are living longer. It is estimated that, while the size of the elderly population in the developed countries will double by the year 2020, in the developing countries there will be a fivefold increase. Thus, for instance, China and India alone can expect to have a further 270 million elderly citizens by that date. This has important implications in terms of the

7

absolute numbers of cataract-blind persons requiring attention over the next two or three decades. Moreover, in many countries in Asia and Africa, it is reported that senile cataract is being seen in 40 to 50 year olds, and sometimes even earlier.

Sex

Although a preponderance of cataract among females has been reported from some countries, this may merely indicate the relatively poorer access of women in general, for one reason or another, to surgical services in those countries. The longer life expectancy of women in some countries also needs to be taken into account.

Possible risk factors

The mechanisms of cataract formation in the human lens are as yet not fully understood. Several studies have focused on epidemiological parameters, such as genetic and environmental influences. Others have been directed towards developmental and molecular biological aspects of the lens and its metabolic and biochemical disorders.

The diversity of the cataractous process, in respect both of morphological appearance and of natural history, has rendered these studies particularly cumbersome and complicated, making it difficult to draw statistically significant and valid conclusions on causal relationships. This is further complicated by the multifactorial pathogenesis of senile cataract.

The possible risk factors for cataract can be grouped under the following headings:

- demographic factors;
- other host factors, including genetic and disease-associated factors;
- environmental factors.

The age of onset of "senile" cataract and its rate of progression also vary widely from one geographical region and climatic zone to another, and various environmental and nutritional or metabolic factors are considered to be responsible for these variations.

8

Demographic factors

The relation of cataract to the aging process has been described earlier (p. 7). The lens participates in the immunocytological and metabolic changes taking place in the body in aging, and the lens changes perhaps reflect these processes.

Host factors

Many drugs and chemicals induce cataract formation under experimental conditions, and some have been associated with cataract formation as a consequence of ingestion or topical absorption when used as medication, e.g., steroids.

Among a number of systemic, metabolic and neurological disorders associated with cataract, diabetes mellitus is perhaps the most important from a public health perspective. After 40 years of age, cataract is commoner in diabetics than in nondiabetics; it is also known that its rate of progression is more rapid in diabetics. With the increase in prevalence of diabetes in many parts of the world, including developing countries, diabetes-related cataract could well be of increasing concern in the future. Altered glucose metabolism in the lens, leading to the accumulation of sorbitol, is considered to be associated with osmotic changes leading ultimately to opacification. Trials are under way to test the efficacy of drugs such as aldose reductase inhibitors in preventing or delaying diabetes-related cataract.

A genetic predisposition to cataract formation seen in consanguineous relatives may also account for the ethnic differences in prevalence found in some epidemiological studies. The underlying cause may be the existence of pharmacogenetic variations that selectively predispose such individuals to environmental cataractogenic influences.

Cataractogenesis has been extensively studied, and it has been suggested that nutrition is one of the many factors that sensitize the lens proteins to change. Differences in nutritional status and dietary composition have been offered as an explanation for the differences in the prevalence and age of onset of cataract in developing as opposed to developed countries.

The coexistence of severe diarrhoea and malnutrition is well recognized. The role of severe diarrhoea *per se* in the causation of acidosis, dehydration and increased plasma urea concentration has been studied extensively. The effects of the osmotic imbalance resulting from rapid dehydration are compounded by those of the raised plasma urea on the lens protein itself through cyanate-induced carbamylation. One or more attacks of severe diarrhoea

9

may be sufficient to sensitize the lens and lead to cataractous change.

If diarrhoea, with its physical and biochemical consequences, is firmly established as a causative or risk factor in cataract, this will open up a whole range of possibilities for preventive interventions against cataract through a primary health care approach, which could be linked with the diarrhoeal diseases control programme.

Environmental factors

The association of cataract with ionizing radiation such as X-rays is well documented, and the role of infrared radiation in glass-blower's cataract is well established. There are also some epidemiological studies which suggest that a positive correlation exists between exposure to near ultraviolet (UVB) radiation (300–400 nm) and chemical and physical changes in lens protein and epithelial cells. A recent study suggests that cortical cataract and extended exposure to UVB are positively correlated.

Conclusions

Senile cataract is an idiopathic disease. While there is an increasing understanding of the biochemical and molecular biological processes taking place in the cataractous lens, it is still not certain whether these are the causes or effects of the process of lens opacification.

The probable multifactorial causation of cataract suggests an interplay of factors, some of which may sensitize the lens components to the noxious influences of others, leading finally to the loss of the normal transparency of the crystalline lens. Further research and a greater understanding of these processes may eventually provide a basis for preventive intervention.

There is thus a need for more epidemiological and basic research which, apart from its scientific and academic interest, could lead to the discovery of a drug or combination of drugs that would make surgical treatment for cataract unnecessary. On the other hand, epidemiological studies may reveal one or more risk factors that could be addressed through appropriate, feasible intervention at the community level. These two complementary research approaches could very well lead to noninvasive treatment and community-based services for the prevention of future cataract blindness, which are likely to be more acceptable, affordable and cost-effective than surgery.

3. Organization of cataract services

The technique for the restoration of vision in patients blind from cataract is well established. It is a relatively simple, safe and effective surgical procedure, in which the cataractous lens is removed. Optical correction is then provided to overcome the ensuing refractive error. The components of a cataract service are thus:

- case-finding and referral;
- surgical services, including follow-up;
- refraction and optical services;
- patient education.

However, access to such services is often woefully poor in most developing countries. Strategies must therefore be evolved to make cataract services physically accessible to those in need of them.

The basic aim should be to deliver cataract surgery services through a primary health care approach. Such an approach would satisfy the essential requirements of acceptability, accessibility, affordability, and scientific soundness. It would also ensure the necessary community involvement and intersectoral action that are essential for the successful outcome of such interventions.

The primary objective of cataract services is to restore vision to the largest number of persons blind from cataract in the shortest possible time, making the best possible use of the existing or potentially available resources at a cost that the community can afford.

Such services should generally be an integral part of national programmes for the prevention of blindness and should at the same time help to develop the permanent infrastructure to deal with the continuing incidence of cataract-related blindness.

The basic steps in managing cataract blindness are as follows:

- assessment of the problem;
- identification of cases;
- creation of an awareness of the problem among the population;
- motivation of the blind to use the services available;
- development of a referral system;
- selection of cases for surgery;
- provision of cost-effective, high-quality surgical services on a mass scale;
- provision of optical correction at an affordable cost;
- monitoring and evaluation.

Assessment of the problem

Assessment of the problem is a prerequisite for planning and setting up the services, and provides baseline data so that the impact of the services can be measured in subsequent evaluations.

Simple and epidemiologically sound data-gathering methods are available either as part of blindness surveys using the eye examination card[1] or through the identification of cataract by community workers trained in eye care. In both these approaches, involving the community will not only enhance awareness of the problem, but also engender and ensure future cooperation when services are organized; this, of course, should be done at the same time as the data are gathered.

A simple and practical method can be used to determine the cataract load in a target area where intervention is planned. The results of such a survey may also be applicable to contiguous or other areas of similar social, economic and ecological character and comparable health infrastructure. As described in Chapter 9, this methodology may be useful in medium-term (2–5 years) evaluation of the performance of cataract services and, more importantly, in determining the extent of the unmet needs so that plans of action can be reformulated and interventions further intensified, as appropriate.

National prevalence studies provide data on the overall prevalence and age distribution of cataract blindness in a country. Such information may be used to determine both the population subgroup to be surveyed and the size of the sample. In the absence of

---

[1] WHO/PBL eye examination record.

survey data, recourse may be had to hospital data or even anecdotal information.

It is unlikely that "clustering" will interfere with the determination of the size of the sample. However, if pockets or villages in the target area are underserved, or specific social, cultural or economic barriers exist in parts of it, the possibility of clustering should be considered in the calculation of the size of the sample. A WHO publication[1] may be consulted for statistical details.

Identification of cases

The objective at the community level is to identify through screening those who are blind and, tentatively, those in whom cataract may be an underlying cause.

The criteria used in recognizing blindness presumably caused by cataract, at the community level, need to be simple. A history of gradual, painless visual loss over a period of years in an older person is suggestive of cataract. The two most relevant objective criteria are:

- visual loss (usually inability to count the fingers of a hand at a distance of 3 metres);
- a grey or white pupil.

The examination does not require expensive equipment; a torch will generally be all that is needed.

Depending on the level of training of the health worker, it may also be possible to include the use of a torch to test the pupillary reaction to light. Such testing should be encouraged whenever feasible.

Creation of an awareness of the problem among the population

One of the difficulties commonly encountered during the detection of individual cases of blindness due to cataract is a lack of awareness, both by the individual and often by key family members, that cataract blindness is curable and that surgery is a safe and effective means of restoring sight.

---

[1] *Methods of assessment of avoidable blindness*. Geneva, World Health Organization, 1980 (WHO Offset Publication No. 54).

The identification at the community level of cases of blindness from cataract makes it possible to motivate those affected to seek surgical treatment, since community health workers, who are usually socially close to members of the community, can communicate information to local populations in general and to affected individuals and their families in particular. This should encourage them to accept and follow the advice given about referral and possible surgical treatment, by overcoming sociocultural, behavioural and other barriers.

Community health workers would need to be prepared for this task by appropriate education and training, which should include, wherever possible, exposure to surgical services, so that the safety and effectiveness of the procedure can be seen at first hand.

Motivation of the blind to use the services available

Creating an awareness among individuals, their families and the community that surgical treatment of cataract is safe and effective is the first important step in promoting acceptance of referral and treatment. Operational research studies in some countries have shown that sociocultural and other barriers can be more easily overcome if people who have undergone successful surgery (aphakics) are used as motivators. In others, the use of trained traditional practitioners as promoters has proved useful.

Transport problems and economic constraints also often need to be addressed. The provision of hospital care and surgical services, including aphakic spectacles, free or at low cost, often enhances compliance.

Development of a referral system

In many countries, blind people detected by the health worker will normally be referred to a health centre or an outreach facility (e.g., eye camp, mobile unit) for further examination before being seen by a cataract surgeon, who selects cases for surgery. At a health centre, skilled or trained personnel are generally available, including nurses with training in eye examination or, in certain situations, more highly qualified staff, including clinical officers and general physicians. At this level, it is generally possible to apply more definitive diagnostic criteria for cataract-related blindness, thus preventing the needless referral for surgical removal of the lens of persons whose blindness is not caused by cataract.

Selection of cases for surgery

The following diagnostic procedures can be performed at a health centre in most circumstances:

- testing of visual acuity in each eye separately;
- examination for projection of light;
- testing of the pupillary reaction to light;
- examination of the appearance of the pupil;
- testing of the red reflex.

In some situations, it may also be possible to measure the intraocular pressure, provided that a tonometer (usually a Schiötz model) is available and that the personnel concerned have been trained in its use. This will prevent the referral of absolute glaucoma patients for surgery—a not infrequent occurrence at outreach facilities.

The equipment required for diagnosis will include an appropriate vision test chart, a torch, a binocular loupe, an ophthalmoscope, and a Schiötz tonometer.

Referral for surgery will depend not only on the patient's ocular status, but also on the place at which surgical services are being provided. It is important that the health centre or other unit providing the services is capable of dealing quickly with the cases referred to it. An overloading of the referral system, leading to undue delays and disappointments for patients and their families, will undermine the credibility of the system and should be avoided. It is therefore necessary to streamline the referral mechanism as far as possible by establishing a recording system for the patients referred and also to provide feedback from the higher levels of eye care to the health workers within the community.

As a routine procedure, a written record or a special card should be provided for each patient referred, stating name, age, place of residence, date and reason for referral. The last of these might be a tentative diagnosis in the broadest terms, which could be useful not only in the evaluation of the performance and competence of the community health worker, but also as an indicator of further training needs.

Feedback from the first referral or higher level should be organized on a continuing basis, e.g., by return of the referral form with a brief description of the action taken, or periodic review of the referral cards during briefing meetings between community health workers and personnel at higher levels.

Provision of cost-effective, high-quality surgical services on a mass scale

To deal effectively with the public health problem of the massive backlog of cataract, it is essential that any large-scale cataract service employs safe and streamlined routines that will ensure quality surgical care. An efficient management system is also essential.

Surgical services for cataract should be an integral part of national programmes for the prevention of blindness, which in turn should be an integral part of the health care system. In underserved communities or in areas where a large cataract backlog already exists, an intensive approach to deal with this backlog may be justified. Such an approach, which should involve the locally available personnel, should aim not only at clearing the backlog, but also at contributing towards the development of the necessary infrastructure that will make the country or region capable of providing eye care services, including cataract surgical services, without outside help in the long term.

4. Therapeutic strategies

The restoration of sight in cataract involves two specific components:

(a) the surgical removal of the cataractous lens;
(b) the correction of the ensuing refractive error (aphakic error).

Choice of technique

The surgical removal of the lens can be effected by either of two basic techniques:

(a) intracapsular cataract extraction (ICCE);
(b) extracapsular cataract extraction (ECCE).

There is general agreement that the safety, speed and simplicity of ICCE under local anaesthesia render it the technique of choice, at present, for mass intervention programmes for senile cataract.

The new microsurgical techniques of ECCE, together with the implantation of an intraocular lens behind the iris, however, afford a level of visual rehabilitation that surpasses that achieved with optical correction with aphakic spectacle lenses. Late posterior segment complications, such as cystoid macular oedema and retinal detachment, are also reported to be marginally fewer than with ICCE. However, these advantages are offset in the context of mass cataract intervention programmes by a number of disadvantages which militate against the universal adoption of ECCE with intraocular lens implantation as a routine technique in such programmes at present.

To begin with, the change to the newer technique would require the retraining of a large number of cataract surgeons in developing countries adept at ICCE. It would also require the provision of operating microscopes, microsurgical instruments, intraocular lenses and other supplies, which are currently far beyond the reach of most developing countries.

Moreover, the greater length of time required for each ECCE compared with ICCE would further reduce the surgical output in terms of the number of cataract operations performed—an important consideration when dealing with the massive cataract backlog.

Following ECCE, secondary cortex formation and clouding of the posterior capsule are not uncommon. The need to deal with this secondary opacification of the posterior capsule in up to a third of the operated eyes within two years, using high-technology equipment such as the Nd:YAG laser, further supports the choice of ICCE with aphakic spectacle correction as the most appropriate technology at present in mass intervention programmes.

The technique of ICCE is described in the Annex (p. 33).

Follow-up procedures

It has already been noted that, depending on local conditions, cataract surgery may be carried out in a variety of settings, including specialized eye hospitals or departments, district hospitals, beds in peripheral hospitals used temporarily by visiting mobile teams, or improvised wards, as in eye camps. In all these varied situations, acceptable standards of operating theatre equipment, aseptic surgical techniques and arrangements for postoperative care are of critical importance in ensuring that good-quality services are provided.

It is vital that the following basic criteria are satisfied for the surgical techniques and in follow-up care:

- the surgical technique must provide good wound closure so as to prevent complications during early mobilization of the patient;
- the patient must be able to comply with the advice provided and receive the postoperative treatment prescribed;
- the patient should normally be available for daily postoperative assessment for a few days, and for a subsequent full examination and provision of spectacles;
- the length of time that the patient is kept in hospital should take into account the socioeconomic situation and the logistic problems existing in the area concerned, and should not be determined solely on the basis of current practice in the developed countries.

Postoperative treatment of the operated eye usually includes topical mydriatics, antibiotics and often corticosteroids. Personnel at the primary health care level may assist in the provision of this treatment, inpatient surveillance and subsequent referral, as necessary.

Monitoring and quality assurance

One of the criticisms repeatedly made of outreach services for mass cataract intervention programmes is that follow-up care is inadequate and quality assurance even less satisfactory. Such observations have in the past detracted from the general usefulness of these services. There is recognition of the need both to ensure safe, high-quality care and for more intensive review of postoperative results through some form of monitoring mechanism. These would enhance the credibility of the system, not only among patients, their families and the community, but also among some of the professionals who have misgivings and reservations about such services.

In some situations, it may be useful to involve community health workers and staff at health centres in the detection and follow-up of possible postoperative complications, such as infection or sudden visual loss.

At all events, the recording of complications during and immediately after surgery, and during the follow-up period, should be an integral part of the system for the provision of cataract surgery. Records should preferably be kept in a systematic and standardized manner, with regular analysis and review to permit identification of specific complications and also to assess the quality of performance of the operating surgeon and surgical team in a particular setting. This would also alert the operating surgeon to any untoward complications, such as multiple postoperative infections resulting from a breakdown in the sterilization routine. It is also important that quality control be carried out independently, preferably by the appropriate professional organizations.

Correction of aphakic refractive error

The resultant refractive error in aphakia can be corrected by one of the following methods:

- spectacle correction;
- contact lenses; this method is not feasible in large-scale

interventions because of both high cost and handling difficulties for the patient;

- intraocular lens implantation; this is not considered further
  here because of the surgical techniques involved;
- refractive corneal surgery; this is still experimental, and is
  available only in highly specialized institutions.

After extraction of the cataractous lens in mass intervention
programmes, therefore, optical correction by spectacles needs to be
prescribed or provided for optimal visual rehabilitation. This is
a formidable problem in many developing countries, given the fact
that spectacles are often hard to find and generally unaffordable,
even if available.

Provision of optical correction at an affordable cost

The provision of aphakic spectacle correction is considered to
be as important as the surgical procedure itself and should receive
special attention. The following preliminary measures may be
adopted to overcome the shortage of aphakic spectacles at an
affordable price.

1. Low-cost, effective technology is available for the local
   assembly of spectacles from locally manufactured or imported
   lenses and spectacle frame components. For this purpose,
   optical workshops, equipped with a simple set of tools for
   surfacing and cutting lenses and fitting them into frames, can be
   established. Standardized spectacle components can be
   imported in bulk to reduce costs. The optical workshop may
   employ two or three trained technicians, and may form part of
   a hospital or eye department, or be run by a local nongovernmental organization.[1] Technicians can usually be trained in
   6–8 weeks. The initial investment required is approximately
   US$ 15 000–20 000, which includes the cost of an initial stock of
   spectacle components. The cost of spectacles produced in these
   optical workshops ranges from US$ 3 to US$ 6 and, if the
   selling price includes a small profit margin, the local assembly
   of spectacles could develop into an economically viable venture.
   In addition, collaboration with ministries of finance and/or

---

[1] *The provision of spectacles at low cost.* Geneva, World Health Organization, 1987.

commerce might enable materials and equipment to be imported at preferential rates of duty, if not duty free.

2. Cheap spectacles may be imported from some countries, such as India, but this requires foreign exchange and high import duties may have to be paid. Although this is an acceptable option on a short-term or interim basis, it does not promote future national self-reliance and is not generally desirable.

3. In countries where there is an existing industry for the production of lenses and frames, it has sometimes been possible to reduce the costs either through bulk purchase or by requesting specially discounted prices on a welfare basis, thus enabling aphakic spectacle components to be assembled and provided for patients who cannot afford them.

4. In some countries the optical industry and opticians can be induced to make spectacles available at reduced prices to deserving individuals. Such a scheme may, however, be undermined by lengthy bureaucratic procedures.

5. The donation of used spectacles by organizations in developed countries is a popular activity. However, the time and effort required in sorting out suitable lenses and frames often detract from the usefulness of such donations, except to a very limited extent for small-scale projects.

The ability to repair and replace aphakic spectacle lenses and frames, where necessary, is of vital importance, and the availability of local workshops to undertake these tasks readily and quickly avoids frustrating delays and is greatly appreciated by the community. The use of standardized frames and lenses would overcome the need to stock a large variety of spares and make repair and replacement easier.

5. Material requirements

Surgical beds and operating-room time

The obstacles to increasing surgical output include the shortage of hospital beds and the limited operating-room time available. These are important issues which must be seen in the context of the competing demands of other disciplines within the health care delivery system.

While the problems of the shortage of surgical beds and their high attendant costs are being solved by providing ambulatory or day surgery (outpatient surgery) in many developed and urban settings, in rural areas of developing countries such approaches are fraught with practical difficulties and certain risks. A compromise approach is to reduce the duration of postoperative hospitalization to the minimum without increasing the risk of avoidable complications. In this context, the proper closure of the wound is important in ensuring quicker patient discharge from hospital.

The problem of limited operating-room time and space can be solved by employing underused operating-theatres in peripheral hospitals, increasing the number of operating tables, within feasible limits, in existing theatres, and setting up makeshift theatres of an acceptable standard, preferably alongside existing facilities.

These approaches will require the provision of additional equipment, surgical instruments and supplies, which are often inadequate even to meet the requirements of the existing limited operation lists. The additional staffing needed if these approaches are adopted is considered in Chapter 6.

Since services may often need to be provided outside the traditional eye care institutions, the organization of such services needs to be worked out in detail so as to ensure both safety and cost-effectiveness.

Surgical supplies and equipment

The existence of an efficient delivery system together with an adequate inventory of surgical supplies and equipment and regular logistic support is of crucial importance if a smooth and uninterrupted surgical turnover is to be achieved. In this context, it is also necessary to ensure that facilities are available or are developed for the rapid maintenance and repair of ophthalmic equipment and surgical instruments, either locally or in a regional or central workshop.

Topical ophthalmic medications and sutures are important requirements, and currently account for a sizeable proportion of the cost of cataract surgery. Innovative approaches are being adopted in some countries to promote local production of low-cost eye medications and sutures, and such approaches should be encouraged and adopted wherever possible. Some nongovernmental organizations have already gained expertise and experience in this area and could assist countries in setting up the necessary facilities, besides providing other supplies and equipment.

6. Personnel

Categories of personnel

The personnel involved in cataract intervention programmes may include:

- (a) community health workers for (i) the identification and referral of patients, (ii) postoperative follow-up, and (iii) community education and motivation;
- (b) ophthalmic nurses and ophthalmic assistants for (i) screening of referred cases, (ii) pre- and postoperative care, (iii) assisting in surgery, and (iv) supervision of primary-level staff;
- (c) cataract surgeons, who may be (i) clinical officers, (ii) ophthalmic medical officers, (iii) general surgeons trained in cataract surgery, and (iv) ophthalmologists.

In most countries where a cataract backlog exists, there is a serious shortage of trained personnel to deal with the problem, and particularly of cataract surgeons. In these countries, a rapid increase in the numbers of such personnel is necessary in order to permit the implementation of large-scale cataract intervention programmes. In a few countries, despite an adequate number of cataract surgeons, their surgical potential, for one reason or another, is seriously underutilized. It is essential in such countries to look into and correct this shortcoming.

In countries where there is a serious shortage of cataract surgeons, there are in general the following four ways of increasing their number:

1. Increase the number of trained ophthalmologists able to undertake cataract surgery. This will require considerable investment in teaching facilities, and the necessary training is expensive and

will yield sufficient numbers only after several years, in view of the length of time required to qualify as an ophthalmologist in most countries. Shorter periods of training, after which a diploma in ophthalmology is awarded, would ensure that adequately trained staff were available more quickly to meet the immediate needs. Such training courses, in which the emphasis would be on cataract surgery skills, should be given particular encouragement and support in order to increase the number of ophthalmologists quickly.

2. Increase the number of cataract surgeons among the ophthalmologists in a country. The underutilization of cataract surgical potential has already been mentioned. It should be possible to involve national ophthalmological societies more fully in cataract intervention programmes by persuading members to play a more active role in cataract surgery by volunteering to work for a time, particularly in rural areas, as part of a mobile team or at a fixed facility such as a district hospital or primary health care centre. Junior ophthalmologists assigned to work in underserved areas for a limited period can be supported and encouraged to perform more cataract surgery.

3. Increase the number of cataract surgeons by training existing general surgeons or medical officers in cataract surgical skills. Some countries have experience of such training over periods ranging from 3 to 12 months. While the duration of training will be determined, among other things, by previous surgical experience, this will not only permit a rapid increase in the number of cataract surgeons in a country but also facilitate their deployment in areas where cataract services are currently inadequate.

4. Train paramedical personnel, such as ophthalmic assistants, to perform cataract surgery. This would be the approach favoured by countries with only a small number of doctors and where legislation permits trained ophthalmic assistants (clinical officers) to perform cataract surgery. Several countries (particularly in Africa) have adopted this approach and found it to give satisfactory results.

These approaches are obviously not generally applicable to all countries and will need to be adapted to each country's particular situation, needs and policies. Some of them will enable the number of people able to perform cataract surgery in a country to be rapidly increased and thus overcome one of the major obstacles to increasing the number of such sight-restoring operations.

25

Teamwork

Cataract surgery, especially as a mass intervention, is a team effort. The complementary nature of the functions of the various members of the team needs to be understood and appreciated. Task-oriented training of all team members should be based on the skills that they need to acquire and in which competence is necessary. The periodic assessment and evaluation of their performance will determine what further education and training they need.

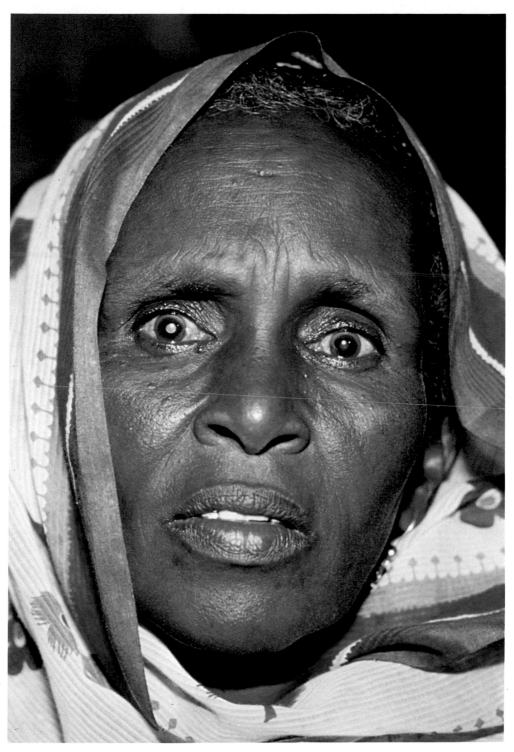

This patient has bilateral senile cataract. The right pupil is densely white (mature cataract), while the left is faintly grey to white in colour from a less developed (immature) cataract.

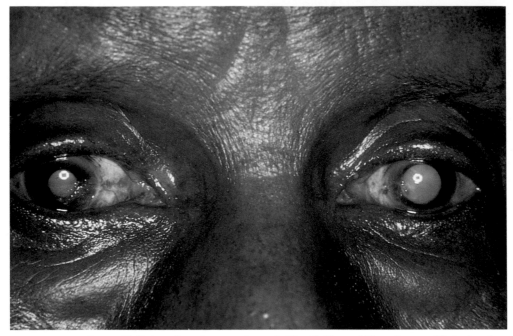

A close-up view of bilateral mature cataract. The left pupil has been dilated prior to surgery. Each cornea shows an abnormality over the inferonasal quadrant. This is climatic keratopathy not directly related to the cataract.

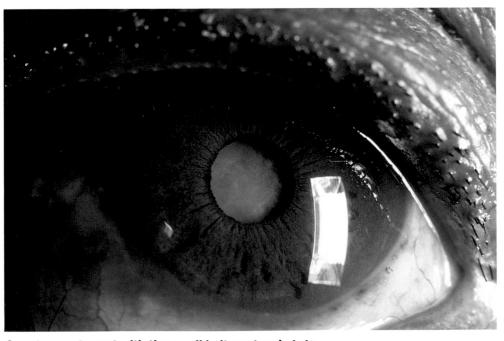

A mature cataract with the pupil in its natural state.

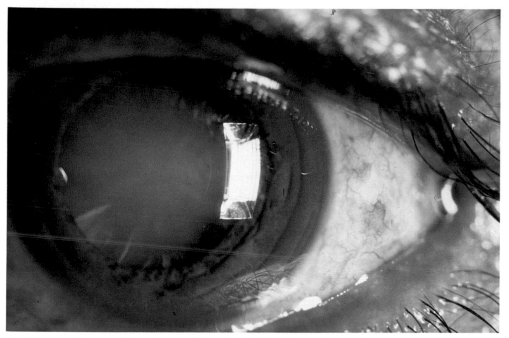

In this eye the pupil has been dilated and the lens shows the spokes of a cortical cataract together with the amber-coloured nuclear changes.

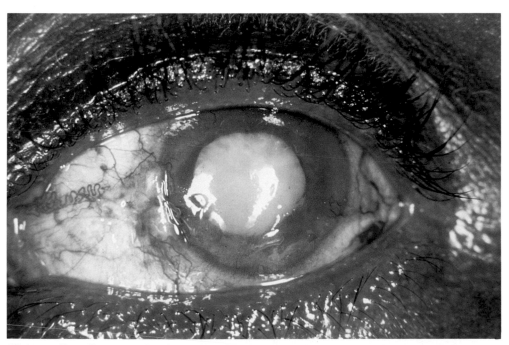

The swollen (intumescent) opaque lens causes the anterior chamber to become shallow and may lead to secondary glaucoma and irreversible blindness.

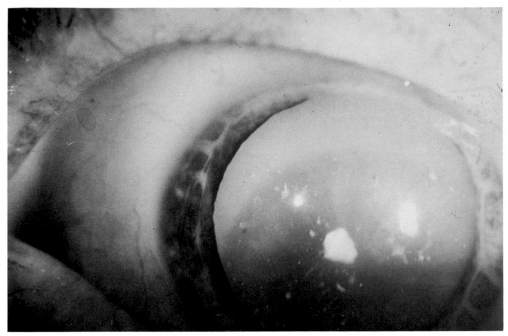

The cortex of this cataract has liquefied (Morganian cataract) and the amber-coloured nucleus is sinking towards the lower pole. Such a lens is more prone to set up a lens-induced inflammation.

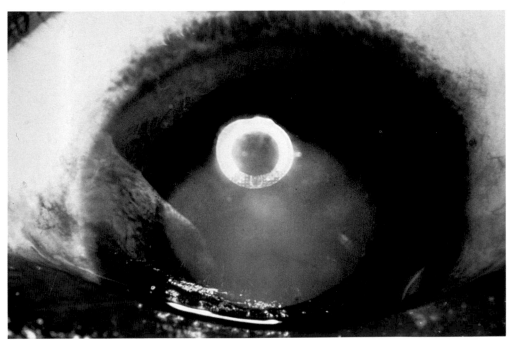

This cataractous lens has subluxated downwards.

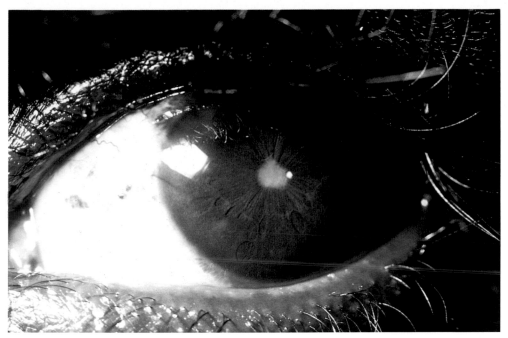

This cataract is the result of earlier uveal inflammation (secondary cataract). The constricted, irregular pupil attached to the lens (posterior synechia) is a tell-tale mark of previous uveitis.

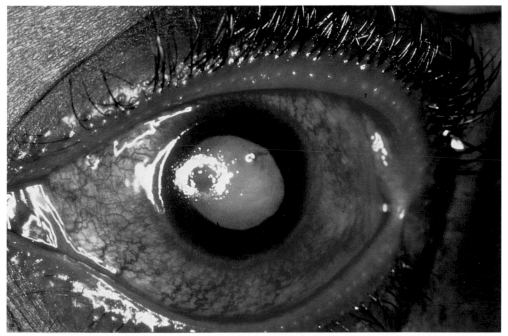

The opacification of this lens is the result of injury (traumatic cataract). The lens is swollen and the eye inflamed. Specialized investigation and treatment are necessary.

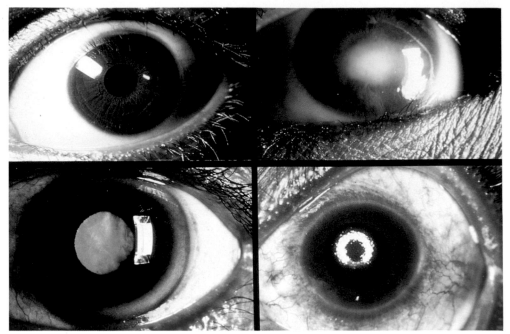

At a community level, cataract should be distinguished from other causes of blindness. Top left: a normal eye; top right: a corneal scar; bottom left: a cataract; bottom right: an eye with chronic open-angle glaucoma (corneal oedema, semidilated, dark pupil (no cataract)). Examination of the cornea, pupil and intraocular pressure will help in the differential diagnosis.

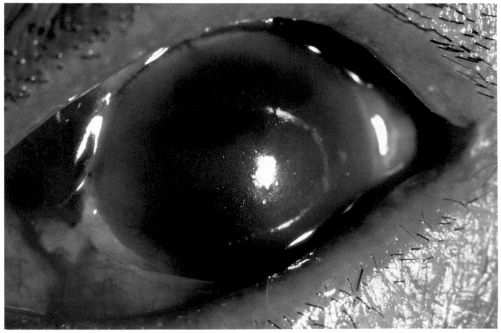

This is an eye following cataract surgery with blood in the anterior chamber (hyphaema). Most cases of hyphaema resolve spontaneously with bed rest and double padding. With adequate wound closure this is an infrequent complication.

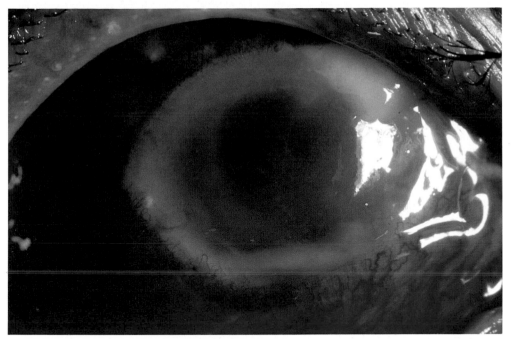

This eye developed postoperative infection (endophthalmitis) a few days after cataract surgery. This is a serious complication requiring urgent and intensive treatment. With careful attention to aseptic technique, it is now rare.

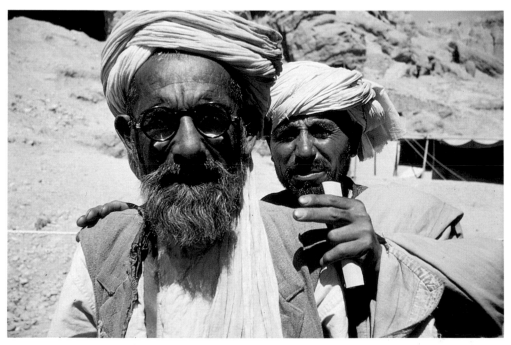

The provision of spectacles following cataract surgery is an important component of cataract intervention services.

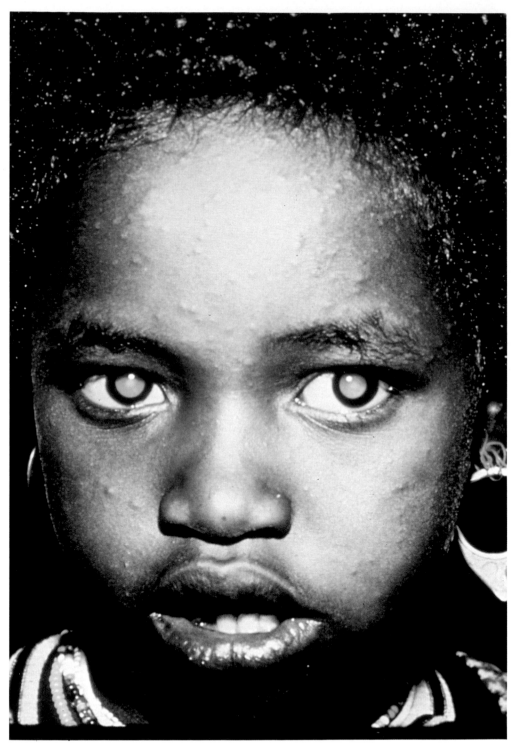

This seven-year-old child has bilateral mature cataract, present from birth (congenital cataract). Its adequate management generally requires a general anaesthetic and specialized treatment facilities.

7. Community participation, role of nongovernmental organizations and coordination with other health programmes

Community participation in eye health activities is essential. Making the community more aware of the problem of cataract blindness is a prerequisite for promoting such participation. The possible role of the community in reducing the burden of cataract should also be stressed. At the same time as the community is encouraged to become involved, it will be helpful to identify the resources available within the community itself to support any proposed activities. Potential resources from outside the community should also be sought. Local service organizations and philanthropic individuals can often be identified and persuaded to provide support, and such benefactors abound in some countries.

Nongovernmental organizations, both national and international, provide technical and financial support to cataract intervention programmes in many areas. In fact, the majority of cataract operations in several developing countries are being carried out with the support of such organizations. In many instances, nongovernmental organizations have been the first to take action in this field, and their example has led to governmental interest, involvement and support.

Nongovernmental organizations and professional societies can also advocate the allocation of resources and the enactment of legislation, where necessary, to ensure quality services. They can support and encourage research and demonstration projects. The education of the public and of members of the medical and allied professions, and participation in the development of standards for diagnosis and treatment are other activities in which they can usefully become involved.

The basic strategy to be adopted by nongovernmental organizations should be to encourage the development of indigenous skills and self-reliance. National resources should be developed gradually in order to take over these activities after support from nongovernmental organizations has been phased out.

Several health programmes are directly concerned with eye health problems, in particular those dealing with the health of the elderly and with rehabilitation, since visual problems, including blindness from cataract, have been identified as a major cause of disability in the elderly. Such disability has serious implications for activities of daily living, and thus has a bearing on the quality of life. Cooperation and collaboration between these programmes at the national level could have a significant, mutually reinforcing and beneficial impact on cataract blindness. Links can also be established between nongovernmental organizations active in these various programmes, so that coordinated action can be planned and carried out with the aim of clearing the cataract backlog.

8. Operational research

Operational research, in the context of cataract intervention programmes, may be defined as the scientific application of analytical methods during planned programme implementation. Its function is to provide decision-makers with the information necessary to enable them to choose the most appropriate course of action to achieve their objectives.

The application of strategies for surgical intervention in cataract depends on several factors, some of which have already been referred to. The delivery of the technology requires not only an efficient system for that purpose, but also a community that is receptive to and accepts the technology and has access to the system.

Operational research addresses the constraints and problems associated with various aspects and phases of the application of the technology and identifies methods and strategies for optimizing the delivery and utilization of cataract services.

While several cataract relief schemes are in place in various developing countries, they are often not very efficient, particularly in terms of surgical output. There are a number of reasons for this, including problems related to the individual, the family and the community, as well as inadequacies in the health infrastructure and limited resources. Operational research, which must clearly be multidisciplinary in character, is often able to disentangle this complex set of interrelated problems and provide practical solutions that make it possible to streamline and optimize services.

Studies of the obstacles to effective community compliance and methods of overcoming them, e.g., by the use of successfully operated patients ("aphakic motivators"), are instances of the application of operational research in cataract surgical programmes.

Demonstration projects for cataract surgery can also be regarded as a form of operational research which aims at developing methods of intervention at the community level to deal with the cataract backlog. Such demonstration projects need to be evaluated in terms both of cost-effectiveness and applicability on the national or regional scale with the limited resources normally available.

Operational research studies should be an integral part of prevention of blindness programmes in general and of cataract relief services in particular so that the best use can be made of the physical, human and financial resources available.

9. Evaluation

Evaluation should form an important and integral part of the operation of cataract intervention services. The objectives set should be expressed in quantitative terms by means of precisely defined indicators, and an appropriate recording and reporting system established so that all the relevant information needed for carrying out the evaluation is available.

Evaluation should focus not only on the surgical output, important though this may be, but also on long-term visual results and complications and on such factors as efficiency, effectiveness and cost. Efficiency implies the assessment of the results achieved by programmes in terms of the efforts made and the resources allocated to attaining the objectives. It takes into consideration issues such as the methods employed, the workforce deployed, the resources used and managerial control.

Determining effectiveness in a cataract intervention programme involves the assessment of how well it has attained its targets, e.g., its contribution to the reduction of the cataract backlog. Cost-effectiveness and cost-benefit analyses also form part of the determination of effectiveness, which may involve specific operational research studies. Cost is of particular importance in view of the limited funding available for such programmes.

The results of short-term evaluations of surgical output, for instance, which should be carried out both regularly and frequently should be shared rapidly with providers of services, so as to guide them in their activities and stimulate and encourage them to increase their efforts.

Long-term evaluation will help in assessing unmet needs and identifying underserved areas. Such evaluation could also usefully include the measurement of the impact of the services, not only on eye health status and well-being, but also in economic terms, wherever feasible. The effect on life expectancy would also be an indicator of the impact of a programme.

In conclusion, the success of cataract intervention programmes in reducing rates of cataract blindness can be assessed in terms of the following:

- *Short-term targets* (0.5–2 years): Number of cataract operations performed and their visual outcome.
- *Short- and medium-term targets* (0.5–5 years): Results of village-level randomized prevalence surveys for cataract blindness in adults over, say, 50 years of age.
- *Long-term targets* (over 6 years): Results of prevalence surveys for cataract blindness as part of definitive blindness survey.

The identification in the course of the evaluation of problems in respect of infrastructure, human resources, community support and resources will assist planners and managers in taking appropriate measures to solve them.

Evaluation of blindness prevention programmes in general, including cataract services, is described elsewhere.[1]

---

[1] *Evaluation mechanisms for programmes for the prevention of blindness.* Unpublished WHO document WHO/PBL/84.9. Available on request from: Programme for the Prevention of Blindness, World Health Organization, 1211 Geneva 27, Switzerland.

Annex

Technique of intracapsular cataract extraction[1]

The surgical technique of choice in mass cataract intervention schemes, for reasons noted earlier, is an intracapsular cataract extraction followed by the provision of spectacles.

Preoperative assessment

The criteria for the diagnosis of cataract requiring surgery are:

- a grey or white pupil;
- the presence of a variably opaque lens as shown by a diminished or absent red reflex;
- visual impairment that interferes with the patient's daily activities (generally considered to be acuity less than 3/60 in the better eye, but may vary according to the patient's visual requirements);
- accurate light projection;
- a pupil reactive to light.

---

[1] Adapted from: Cook, J. et al., ed. *General surgery at the district hospital*. Geneva, World Health Organization, 1988. The various stages of the operation and the complications that may arise are described only very briefly. It must be borne in mind that individual surgeons may have their own preferences regarding surgical technique and specific medication. Reference may be made to textbooks of ophthalmic surgery for more detailed descriptions of both operative techniques and the management of postoperative complications.

The surgeon must establish, as far as possible, that (*a*) there is no underlying pathology in the optic disc or retina that would militate against a successful visual outcome and that (*b*) intraocular pressure is not raised at the time of surgery.

General examination

This should include a medical check-up and treatment if necessary for diabetes mellitus, hypertension and any bleeding diathesis. Periocular foci of infection, such as an infected lachrymal sac, would be a contraindication to surgery.

Preoperative preparation

The following steps should be taken:

1. Wash the patient's face on admission.
2. Apply eye drops (0.5% chloramphenicol) or eye ointment (1% tetracycline) every 8 hours, starting 24 hours prior to surgery.
3. Instil a mydriatic.
4. Administer premedication (promethazine 25 mg and/or diazepam 10 mg) orally one hour before surgery. Oversedation should be avoided, particularly in older patients, and such premedication may be omitted in some instances.
5. If required, give acetazolamide 250 mg orally 8 hours and 2 hours before surgery.

Anaesthesia

Retrobulbar block

Retrobulbar block is effected by injecting 2.5 ml of 2% (20 g/litre) lidocaine into the cone formed by the rectus muscles. With the patient supine, palpate the orbit of the eye to locate the lower outer border. Introduce a 23-gauge, 2.8 cm needle vertically at this point (Fig. 1A). Penetrate the skin and then the orbital septum; resistance will be encountered as the needle passes through each of these two layers. Once the tip of the needle is lying below and behind the globe, angle the needle in the direction of the junction between the roof and the medial wall of the orbit

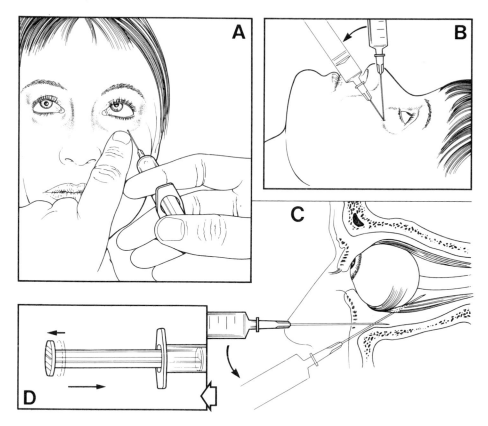

Fig. 1. Retrobulbar block. Palpating the lower orbital margin and introducing the needle perpendicularly, close to its outer corner (A); angling the needle towards the junction of the roof and the medial wall of the orbit behind the globe (B, C); drawing back the plunger as the needle penetrates the muscle (D).

(Fig. 1B, C). Introduce it further and penetrate the muscle layer, which will be indicated by a slight resistance. Draw back the plunger of the syringe (to make sure that the tip of the needle is not in a vein) (Fig. 1D) and inject the local anaesthetic. It should flow freely. Resistance may mean that the tip of the needle is lodged in the sclera, in which case move the tip of the needle slightly from side to side until it is disengaged.

If the needle has accidentally entered a vein, resulting in haemorrhage and a rapid swelling of the orbit, abandon the procedure. Delay the operation for at least one week, after which it can be performed with the patient under either another retrobulbar block or, preferably, general anaesthesia.

35

Facial block

To produce facial block, 2–3 ml of 2% (20 g/litre) lidocaine is injected into the area 2 cm in front of and below the tragus of the ear (Fig. 2).

Topical

Topical anaesthesia can be achieved with one drop of 0.5% tetracaine (5 g/litre) or similar drug in the conjunctival sac 15 minutes before surgery.

Intermittently massage the globe over the closed lids for about a minute to decompress the orbit and prevent forward movement of the vitreous body during surgery.

Surgical field preparation

Clean the ocular adnexa and face with 1% cetrimide and drape the surgical field with sterile towels. Irrigate the surface of the eye and fornices with sterile saline.

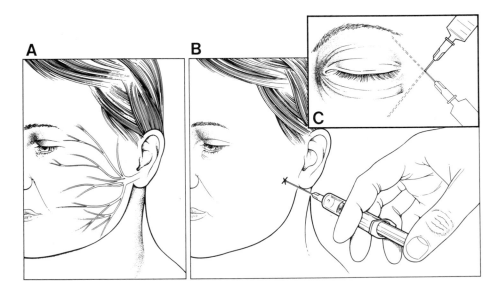

Fig. 2. Facial block. The facial nerve and its branches (A); injecting local anaesthetic in front of and below the tragus of the ear (B); as an alternative, injecting local anaesthetic along the orbital margins (C).

Surgical step 1

Objective

To retract the lids during surgery.

Method

Introduce a speculum such as a light wire lid speculum. This may be combined with an upper lid suture using 4/0 cotton thread to ease closure of the lid over the globe after surgery.

Surgical step 2

Objective

To control depression of the eyeball.

Method

Place a bridle suture (3/0 thread) under the superior rectus muscle. With toothed forceps, grasp the conjunctiva at the edge of the cornea in the region of 12 o'clock[1] and turn the eye down. With another pair of forceps, grasp the superior rectus tendon near its insertion and pass the suture under the tendon (Fig. 3B). Clip the looped suture to the drape.

Surgical step 3

Objective

To expose the limbal corneoscleral area for making the incision.

Method

Make a conjunctival flap. A fornix-based flap is preferred. Incise the conjunctiva at the limbus from 9 to 3 o'clock (Fig. 3C)

---

[1] To interpret references to 12 o'clock, 9 o'clock, etc., imagine a clock face superimposed on the patient's cornea, with 12 o'clock nearest the patient's supraorbital margin.

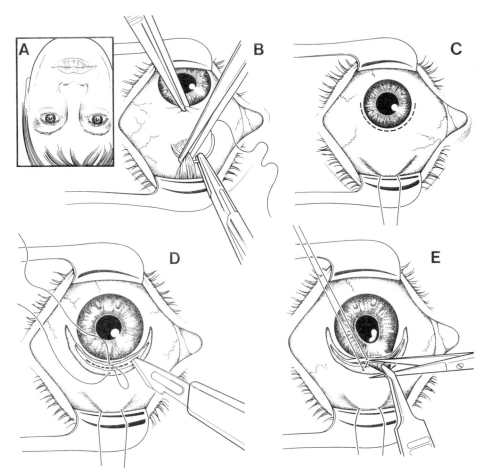

Fig. 3. Intracapsular extraction of cataract. Position of the patient (A, as seen by the surgeon at the head of the table); turning the eye down and passing a suture beneath the superior rectus tendon (B); site of conjunctival incision (C); incising along the limbus and inserting a suture across the groove (D); excising a small piece of the iris (E).

and separate it from the limbus with conjunctival scissors. Achieve haemostasis by cauterizing bleeding points with a hot-point cautery.

Surgical step 4

Objective

To open the anterior chamber.

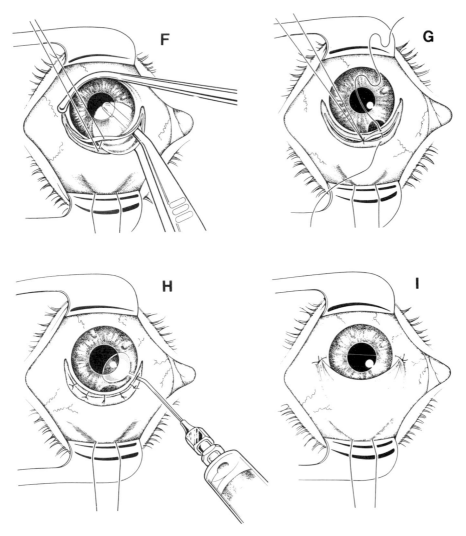

Fig. 3. Intracapsular extraction of cataract (*continued*). Extracting the lens (F); tying the preplaced suture and inserting further sutures to close the corneo-scleral incision (G); reforming the anterior chamber by injecting a small air bubble (H); drawing the conjunctival flap down over the wound and anchoring it (I).

Method

Make an incision perpendicular to the surface of the globe from about 10 to 2 o'clock along the limbus, cutting through one-half to two-thirds of the depth of the corneoscleral tissue.

Insert an 8/0 thread suture across the groove at 12 o'clock and loop it aside (Fig. 3D). Open the anterior chamber with a No. 11 blade or keratome through the groove at the 12 o'clock position and extend the corneoscleral section along the groove using corneal scissors.

Surgical step 5

Objective

To make an opening in the iris.

Method

While an assistant lifts the cornea gently with the looped corneoscleral suture, grasp the iris at its base at 12 o'clock with iris forceps. Gently withdraw the iris outside the incision and excise a small piece at its base with iris scissors to form a peripheral iridectomy (Fig. 3E).

Surgical step 6

Objective

To remove the cataractous lens from the eye.

Method

While the assistant gently lifts the cornea as before, introduce the closed intracapsular forceps into the eye. Grasp the anterior capsule of the lens with the forceps near the 6 o'clock position. Using counterpressure on the outside at the inferior limbus with a muscle hook or lens extractor (Fig. 3F), move the lens from side to side to break the zonules and slide it out of the eye. A cryoextractor is preferable and, when available, can replace the intracapsular forceps.

Surgical step 7

Objective

To restore the anterior chamber.

Method

Reposition the iris by stroking it clear of the incision and back into the eye, using an iris repositor. Intraocular irrigation with sterile saline may be necessary at this time if pigment deposits or blood are left in the anterior chamber.

Tie and cut the preplaced suture. Insert at least four additional 8/0 thread sutures at regular intervals, tie and cut—this closes the corneoscleral incision (Fig. 3G). The anterior chamber may now be reformed by injecting a small quantity of sterile air through a fine cannula attached to a syringe (Fig. 3H).

Surgical step 8

Objective

To reposition the conjunctival flap.

Method

The superior rectus bridle suture is removed by dividing one loop of the suture close to the conjunctiva and withdrawing it. The conjunctival flap is then drawn down over the closed corneoscleral wound and anchored, if necessary, by two sutures at the 3 o'clock and 9 o'clock positions using 8/0 thread (Fig. 3I).

Surgical step 9

Objective

To administer prophylaxis against infection.

Method

Inject 20 mg of gentamicin subconjunctivally near the inferior fornix. Crystalline benzylpenicillin 12 mg (20 000 units) may be used instead of gentamicin. Place chloramphenicol 0.5% eye drops or tetracycline 1% eye ointment in the conjunctival sac.

Draw the upper lid over the globe, and strap the lid suture to the skin over the cheekbone. Strap a sterile dressing over the closed eye and apply a protective shield. It is sometimes necessary to put a simple bandage over this dressing.

Postoperative follow-up

The general principles with regard to postoperative follow-up have been outlined earlier. Specific after-care includes the following:

1. *24 hours after surgery*: first postoperative change of dressing, with inspection of the eye and instillation of antibiotic, mydriatic and steroid eye drops as indicated.
2. *Daily*: dressing with the above medication as necessary for 5 days.

Patients are usually discharged from hospital on the fifth day, and are generally seen at 2 weeks to have the sutures removed and at 6 weeks for glasses to be prescribed. A further postoperative visit is scheduled at 6 months.

Complications

The following complications may be associated with planned ICCE.

Complications of anaesthesia

The most important is retrobulbar haemorrhage, which always requires postponement of elective surgery.

Intraoperative complications

These may include the following:

(a) Inadvertent rupture of the lens capsule: this converts the operation into an extracapsular procedure. The lens nucleus is removed with capsule forceps, a sharp hook or vectis, and the remaining lens cortex is washed out by irrigation with sterile saline; ensure that no cortical or capsular material is trapped in the wound.
(b) Vitreous loss during surgery: this can often be prevented by taking care to avoid undue pressure on the globe from a tight lid, speculum or other instrument. If vitreous loss does occur, vitrectomy must be carried out using the "open sky" technique, and the wound and anterior chamber cleared of all vitreous material. The anterior chamber is reformed with air.
(c) Expulsive haemorrhage: this is a serious complication which is not generally amenable to treatment.

42

Postoperative complications

These may include the following:

(a) Shallow anterior chamber: this may be the consequence of a leaking wound resulting from inadequate wound closure. Application of a pressure pad and bandage for 48 hours is often all that is necessary, but it may occasionally be necessary to place additional corneoscleral sutures preferably under general anaesthesia. An air bubble behind the iris may cause a shallow chamber which may be corrected, e.g., by fully dilating the pupil with atropine 1% drops.

(b) Hyphaema: this is usually transient and self-limiting. If it is severe, double patching and bed rest should be prescribed, until the bleeding stops.

(c) Iris incarceration or prolapse: this is nearly always the consequence of poor wound closure, but occasionally the patient may traumatize the eye. Reposition or excision of the iris and resuturing of the corneoscleral wound will be necessary.

(d) Infection (endophthalmitis): this is potentially the most serious postoperative complication of all as it can lead to varying degrees of visual loss, including irreversible blindness. With proper theatre preparation and aseptic technique, it is now a rare complication. However, if it does occur it is important that it be identified early and treated energetically as an emergency. Wherever possible, the patient should be referred to a centre with better facilities for microbiological examination and sophisticated techniques such as vitreous tapping or vitrectomy.

(e) Late postoperative complications: these include cystoid macular oedema, aphakic glaucoma, and aphakic retinal detachment. A description of their diagnosis and management is beyond the scope of this manual, and reference should be made to specialized texts.

49465